THE WEIGHT LOSS SECRET THAT IS FREE

A weight loss incentive and motivation to promote a lifelong healthy body and mind!

By

Minister Deborah Ross

ISBN-13: 978-1512062793

ISBN-10: 1512062790

End Times Publishing, 2015

Printed in the United States of America

Liability Disclaimer

By reading this book, you assume all risks associated with using the advice given below, with a full understanding that you, solely, are responsible for anything that may occur as a result of putting this information into action in any way, and regardless of your interpretation of the advice.

You further agree that our company cannot be held responsible in any way for the success or failure as a result of the information presented in this book. It is your responsibility to conduct your own due diligence if you intend to apply any of our information in any way.

Terms of Use

You are given a non-transferable, "personal use" license to this book. You cannot distribute it or share it with other individuals.

Also, there are no resale rights or private label rights granted when purchasing this book. In other words, it's for your own personal use only.

Contents

Contents 5

Dedication 7

Introduction 9

Chapter One Skinny is a State of Mind 13

Chapter Two Be Transformed 17

Chapter Three Rid Yourself of Old Mindsets 21

Chapter Four Renew Your Mind..................25

Chapter Five Peace of Mind 29

Chapter Six Word and Mind Power 33

Chapter Seven Mind Games 37

Chapter Eight Mind Over Matter.................. 41

Chapter Nine Made Up Mind.........................45

Chapter Ten A Green Mindset.......................49

Chapter Eleven Masculine Mind 55

Chapter Twelve Be Aware, Be Mindful..........61

Conclusion.. 71

Kingdom Keys to Meditate Upon 73

Prayer 75

About the Author..79

Resources 81

Dedication

I am truly grateful to God who has blessed me and given me grace to use every gift and talent for the uplifting and expansion of the Kingdom of God.

It is my testimony to declare that, "if it had not been for the Lord on my side", through the journeys of life, I would not be here today. I stand as His chosen and elect for such a time as this.

I am thankful for all the support of my son, Anthony with great love, my family and the members of Kingdom Life Ministries International. My pastor, Dr. Diane Clark and Minister Terri B. Jones gave of their time and experience to make this project a success. May the Lord bless every one for their love and continued support.

Shalom!

Introduction

My goal has always been to exhort and give encouragement to the Body of Christ. Sometimes that can be as simple as saying, I love you or by sending a written card to someone. It definitely helps to know that you are not alone. I am thankful for all the support I have received in my journey through life.

Perhaps my most difficult journey has been the road of health and wellness. If you were like me, and have a history of losing weight, then gaining it right back, there is help. Now is the time to make a decision. Change your mind and change your life!

You can start a new season of growth and productivity. In you, is the ability to "create" new life!

Beloved of God, I had tried almost every diet and weight plan possible, but to no avail. I was always trying to lose weight. The difference now, is that I am aligning myself with the Word of God that promises good health to His people.

III John 3:2 says *"Dear friend, I pray that you may enjoy good health and that all may go well with you, even as your soul is getting along well."* NIV.

I decided to give the Word of God reign. It is the foundation of life and I needed new life. The Word is medicine; it is health to your bones. It will assist you in the battle of overindulgence and poor eating habits. It definitely worked for me.

You can do it also! Through Christ, you can resist temptation and walk in a new life of victory. You can stop with condemning yourself and be free and at liberty.

As you read "The Weight Loss Secret that is Free", it will break you free from every chain and shackle. No more insecurities; the Lord validates you. You will finally be able to be open again as you come out of hiding; let the root be exposed, and become healed.

He's changing us from glory to glory. Let Him change you from carnality to divinity. It is a process, but stick with it. Remember, you can do all things through Christ, who is your strength. You have every tool you need to be successful and to be victorious. I agree with you! Now, let's get started!

Chapter One
Skinny is a State of Mind

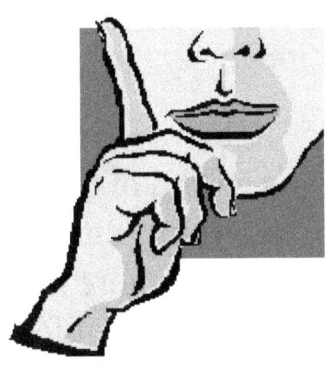 In my mind, I see myself as a beautiful, bold, and attractive woman. He, Christ, beautifies the meek with salvation (Psalms 149: 4). I am the temple whose Gate is called Beautiful (Acts 3:2). The new "60 is 40" woman is what I'm striving for. No hormonal aging (decrease hormone production as you age, especially those that maintain youth and vitality) for me! The Word permeates my body! He renews my strength as the eagle (Psalms 103:5). I am a fruitful bough! My leaf does not wither and my fruit remain! That's me, a woman full of vim and vigor.

Then I look in the mirror. Ok! Who is that person? Where did she come from and where am I? Sounds familiar? Well, the good news is that she's there, just under some layers. So, how do I reclaim or better yet, make myself into this new divine creation?   It definitely will take much divine intervention? I can do it and so can you! Phil 4:13 states: "I can do all things through Christ that strengthens me". Remember that, Greater is He that is in you. You are not alone. He, Christ, supports you. He's got your back! He agrees with you for life and longevity.

Well...here's the skinny (the 411 for the younger ladies). Actually, let's get rid of the word skinny.   It brings to mind, thin, emaciated bodies, fad diets, lettuce, lettuce and more lettuce and always being hungry. That is not the life God has planned for you. He wants you to have an abundant life! The goal is a much healthier and stronger you!

What's healthy for you?   Not what some magazine, multi-media, or Hollywood tells you. Do you have a personal trainer or chef? Most of us don't! You have something most of them don't. You have a relationship with a risen Christ who is concerned about you (II Peter 1:3). He is concerned about those things that pertain to your life and godliness. The whole you! That's body, soul, and spirit.

What is necessary to make you feel better? Let's find out! Each person is different; your body responds differently to certain foods. Knowing how yours work, will assist you in acclimating to your new lifestyle. Let's just clear our minds now from the torment of trying to achieve size 6 or 8. Yea, freedom, freedom! Feels great doesn't it? You can be a healthy BBW (Blessed Beautiful Woman)!

Chapter Two
Be Transformed

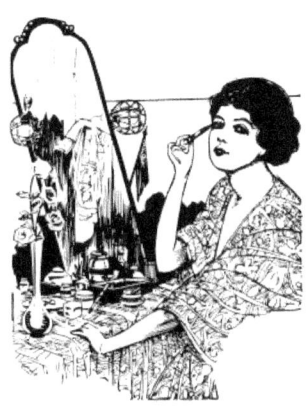 The first thing you must do, of course, is to commit. Make up your mind to follow through, no matter what. I can remember one day looking in the mirror and not liking what I saw. Talk about self-esteem issues. I was uncomfortable in my own skin. Of course, being 260 plus pounds was not good. I knew I was pre-disposed for diabetes. My life style had to change. Change your mind, the rest will follow.

You must speak and think positive to be victorious. You have the mind of Christ! Start declaring that your mind is free from those desires that are not healthy for you. No more self-defeating night binges when you are lonely. Okay?

Christ was victorious in every area of life. So can you! Whenever a situation arose, he always inquired of the Father; he prayed and asked for help. He received strength to help him to persevere and finish his course. He will be right there with you also to assist you to finish your course. Meditating on the Word will keep you motivated as you embark on your "get healthy" journey.

Change starts in the mind. Romans 12: 1-2 tells us to be transformed by the renewing of your mind. Make up your mind not to accept the status quo, and began to see food differently. Not as a panacea for what ails and troubles you, but for nourishment and strength for the body. Our body, which is Christ's temple, is His abode. We must take care of it. Poor eating habits keep us in poor health. It's your season to make that change!

Here are some scriptures to promote your transformation. Your prayer is that the word will become engrafted on the tables of your heart (Psalms 1:2). Meditate on it, think on it, and the Word will begin to distract you from food and your problems and begin to focus on God's love and grace.

Mattew 8:34...".Whosoever will come after me, let him or her deny himself (discipline himself), take up his cross and follow me."

18

Proverbs 13:25...".The righteous eat to the satisfying of his soul, but the belly of the wicked shall want (never satisfied, consumed by lust)."

Proverbs 25:27-28..."It is not good to eat much honey: He that hath no rule over his own spirit is like a city that is broken down, and without walls"

If you were like me, you grew up being told, "Eat your food, there are starving children in Africa" or not eating meant that you were not thankful. So, I ate. Back then, in my day, we worked from sun up to sun down, in the fields of North Carolina that I grew up in. Believe me when I say, "I didn't worry about calories"! I burned up the mega caloric count of beans, fat back, fried chicken, biscuits, candy and cake and other traditional southern soul foods.

Now, it's different. The workforce today, mostly, does not perform heavy manual labor. Technology advances has lessen the need for muscles. Work is sitting at a computer for hours for most of us. We are not in labor intensive work fields. We sit in air-conditioned rooms at our desk and consume coffee, cookies, candy, and doughnuts to our heart's content. The kilo-calories mount up. It takes 3500 calories to make a pound and burning up (metabolizing) 3500 calories to lose a pound. Calorie counting and weighing food just drives me crazy.

I do believe that making healthy choices and watching portions will help to achieve the goal.

No matter the cultural or ethnicity, there is a growing problem of disease and poor health because we are consuming too much sugar, starch, fats, and empty calories that provide no nutritional value. We have become a sluggish and unproductive in our minds and bodies.

Diabetes, obesity, and high blood pressure steadily increase as we eat our way to an early death. Our children are following our example and Juvenile diabetes is on the rise. We have become a nation of overeaters yet physically weak people. Let's change that percentage and let's start to live! The goal is a healthier YOU!

I have worked as a health care professional for over 25 years and can attest to the damage of what a poor eating lifestyle can do. It hit's even closer to home. My mother and four siblings have did from diabetic complications and other related diseases. It is a matter of life and death for me. I choose Life!

Chapter Three

Rid Yourself of Old Mindsets

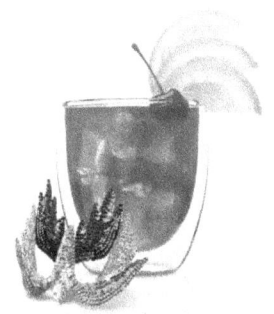

Any conflict, controversy, or battle always begins in your mind. Once making the decision for change and betterment, stick to it. If it's to be, you have to initiate the process.

What's in you ladies? Christ is in you, He's your hope! We have the mind of Christ! He lives in us, so He will empower and enable us to prevail and persevere. We are exhorted to let this mindset to be in us. You can do it!

Know Thyself! Whatever your weakness or weaknesses, you can be strong. You can fortify those areas by changing your mindset. Now, let's set the course. Ok. Get real! The process may take some time. Remember, patience is a virtue. Be honest with yourself! What led to you being in this state? What is the root cause of your over indulgence? When did food become the panacea for all your woes, discontents, and troubles? Will you take the time to be honest with yourself? "To thy own self be true". Pull off that old mindset. Come clean! Admit that it's not hunger that's making you eat more. It is all that sorrow and grief. It is past hurts and offences. Say goodbye to all those disappointments and say hello to a new perspective.

Think about it! When you felt lonely or lost or unloved, that extra cookie or chips was a temporary fix to your dilemma. Eating activates the pleasure zones in our brain. The brain releases endorphins, which gives you a "high". It lets you feel good for a short time. So, instead of casting our cares on Jesus, our burden bearer, we decide to do it ourselves. We eat and eat to fill the voids and empty places in our lives. We are not satisfied. My demise was chocolate chip cookies, pasta, and breads. Yummy!

I confess, I am still challenged in these areas. There is not a chocolate anything I do not like, but there is one thing that is different. I have more discipline! Instead of the whole bag, I stop at two, ok, three. It's unrealistic to think you will never eat your favorites again. It's all about your new soon to become friend, MODERATION! Moderation lets you eat what you like, but with discipline. You take a few bites of that chocolate cake and put down the fork. Instead of the cake, eat a protein bar, have a V8, or better still have a five minute power walk. Drink some lemon water and wait five more minutes. Meditate on a scripture. Wow!

You are getting there!

Chapter Four
Renew Your Mind

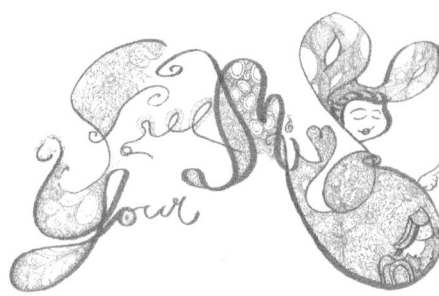 You don't need a fast weight loss scheme or a new diet. You need your mind and perception of you to change. That's seventy five percent of the battle. Be transformed by the renewing of your mind. What renews, refreshes, regenerates and rejuvenates? The living Word! The Word will help me lose weight? Yep! I am a witness. The more I thought positive and inspiring thoughts, the lesser the cravings I had. Truth! If we meditate on it, chew on it, eat it, it will become a part of us that fulfills both naturally and spiritually (Psalms 1:2).

Next, Get a Partner! Be Accountable! James 5:16 tells us, *"Confess your faults one to another and pray for one another, that ye may be HEALED!"* As you are tempted to eat those things that are not profitable for your body, you will have another source of strength. If two shall agree (Matt 18:19). Get a friend; get your husband or a loved one, anyone who will help to keep you moving forward.

The enemy sends these desires, these temptations (James 1:12-15) because you belong to Jesus. If he can handicap you from fulfilling your purpose, he will. Satan doesn't care what methods he uses, just the results. Resist Him! Jesus told Satan, "that man or mankind does not live by bread alone, but by every Word that comes from the mouth of God (Matt 4:4).

I am sure that you no longer want to be under the control of your appetite. The goal is to change from a carnal mentality to a kingdom mentality. You will be changing your body from a carbohydrate desiring one to a green/protein desiring one. Let the Word fill your empty places.

Can I tell you, the next step? Repentance! Once you acknowledge that you missed the mark, and confess. God forgives! If you confess your faults, He is faithful and just to forgive them and cleanse you from all unrighteousness (I John 1:9). Pride will tell you that everyone eats. You might say, "I love to eat. I like food". The spirit of error will have you justify the spirit of gluttony, surfeiting, and overindulgence. Don't let the enemy use food as a tool against yourself.

You are important and you are valuable. You have worth!

You must identify these strongholds, pull them down and dig up the root cause whether, physiological, psychological, or spiritual damage. These things have become strongholds as you have habitually given in to the spirit of lust. I guess you might say, "That's a strong word, lust; but lust of the eye, lust of the flesh, and pride of life are tools the enemy uses to keep you captive".

Forgive yourself! No condemnation! The spirit of life in Christ Jesus has made you free from the law of sin and death (Rom 8:1-3). Sometimes, we are judged by what we eat or drink and conversely, what we don't eat or drink. God is your validation! Follow Him! He loves you and wants you to be YOU!

You can start to feel good about yourself again. Take this time to do something for you. You are deserving of love. Love you! When you look in the mirror, don't see the old you; imagine the new person that is confident and outgoing. I actually went in a shell and hid myself as I increased in weight. I was ashamed and my self-esteem had plummeted. One day, I decided no more! Almost weighing 260 pounds was not for me. I looked at me and I became the responsible for my condition.

Chapter Five
Peace of Mind

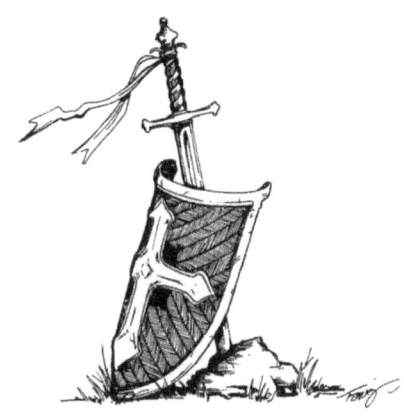

It's on! The battle begins! Whatsoever you bind in Heaven is also bound in earth. Whatsoever you loose in heaven is loose in earth (Matthew 16:19, 18:18). You must take authority over your domain. You are King! The word of a King has power. You have what you say! There is power in the tongue. Speak health, soundness, wellbeing, and temperance in your life. Ask for discipline in this area of your life. Begin to come in agreement with God's plan for you. You will find peace!

The word tells us if we keep our minds on Him, He will keep us in perfect peace (Isa. 26: 3). Perfect peace is the peace that Christ gives you, no matter the circumstance or problem. The peace of God passes all understanding and keeps your heart and mind. You can be confident that He will bring you through whatever He has prepared for you. You must declare and decree! The word is nigh and in your mouth. Speak! Loose the captivity of your spirit, Daughters! Be Free!

According to the power invested in you through Jesus Christ of Nazareth, Bind the spirit of Overindulgence, Gluttony, Lust, and Desire in the Name of Jesus. Then loose the spirit of Temperance, Self-control, and Discipline. Get a prayer partner and come in agreement to start the change in your life.

So, let's forget the pills and such and let's start working on you. You need to like you! What? Every time you say things like, "I'm so fat, I'm ugly, my nose is too big, or I'm too short or too tall", you are decimating you! Psalms 139:14 tells you that, *"you are fearfully and wonderfully made. Marvelous are your (God's) works."* So every time you are negative or speak out of your emotions, (things we say have spirit, they have life or death), you tear down another layer in the walls of your self-esteem. So let's reverse that. God declares that you, You Look Marvelous! Again, I repeat: You have worth! You are valuable! Believe the Lord, not the Hype!

You are a Precious Jewel! It's time to come out of hiding. It's time to come out of your comfort places. It really is a defense mechanism. You reject you, so others cannot reject you. You are not fearful, but valiant! You are not defeated! You are an overcomer! He causes you to triumph and have good success!

Chapter Six

Word and Mind Power

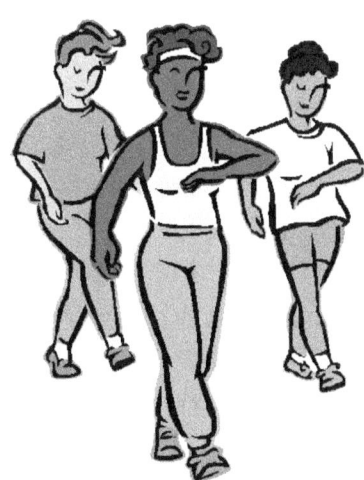Job 23:12 tells us, *"to Esteem the Word more than necessary food"*. See the difference. Food takes a back seat to the Word which gives life and health. It would not hurt to start denying yourself of things that are not healthy for you. I'm not saying to go on a fast, but a gradual letting go of the extra caloric input. It is known that to lose weight, you must decrease calories and/or increase your exercise.

Depending on your health or other factors, you will be able to decide what is best for you! It is all about you right now! There are varied and new weight loss programs and methods, but I do believe if you use the Word as your foundation, it will help you during the times of temptation, when you just got to have that fix.

The prayer is for Moderation coupled with a full helping of Temperance, Self-control, and Discipline. Remember, you didn't get that way overnight and you will not lose it overnight. If weight lost is steady, you are less hap to regain it. All the money I have spent in the pursuance of an image that society says I have to have to be successful would probably feed many hungry children. All the pills, wraps, and starvation would not have been needed if I had trusted God.

In every situation of my life, I needed to stand on His word and believe. I took care of everyone else and let myself go. I know you can relate. You become what you do and not who you are. No longer let food be your "reward". Get out of the house! Change your environment. Walk it out! The reward is worth the time and effort. This is for you!

You are not possessed! You are the Beautiful temple (II Cor. 6:16). I know sometimes you feel that you are a" Little House of Horrors and there is a thing inside you saying, "Feed me, Seymour. Feed me". That's just your carnal man trying to gain control. It is your emotions trying to rule you. You have the power; put the tormenter and his imps out of your domain! The prayer of Binding and Loosing is what needed in this area.

Thank God for Jesus who always causes you to triumph in Him. Satan wants to destroy your temple (Christ lives in you); Satan wants to abort the purpose and plan of God in your life. He thought crucifying Jesus would stop the plan of God. (If he had known, they would not have crucified Him, (II Cor. 2:8). He cannot stop you either! Keep going!

The adversary wants you to be weak and powerless, so you cannot be" fit" and ready for service to God. When you are sick, tired, and unhealthy, you cannot perform in the Excellency of Christ. It affects your job, your home, the work of the ministry, and it affects you. It's all about sabotaging and hindering the purpose for you being here in earth.

How many of you have the enemy told, "That you don't fit in the Body of Christ or that you have nothing to offer just because you don't look like the presumed package? Don't be caught up in outward adorning, it's what's inside (1 Peter 3:3-4) that counts. The real you being validated and at peace; that's what is important.

You are much more than what meets the eye! Beauty is only skin deep, but ugly (the heart is deceitful and wicked) is to the bone. The Lord is your husband! You are Beulah and He delights in you (Isa 62:4). He is the health of your countenance. He gives life and wants you to be your best.

Chapter Seven
Mind Games

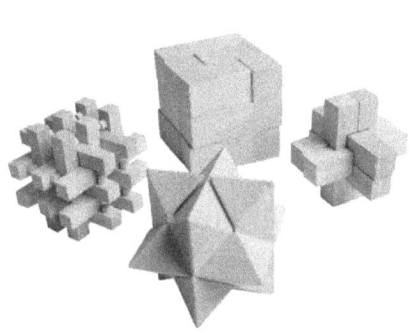 Remember, the carnal man or mind is always at enmity with the spiritual man. When we would do good, evil is always present (Romans 7:13-25). He is always working to make us miss the mark. Use your sword! It's in your mouth! Bind, then Loose. Resist him steadfast in the faith... Your battle is a spiritual one, not a fleshly one. The enemy comes to kill, steal, and destroy, but you overcome by your testimony and the blood of the Lamb. As you resist the enemy of your soul and submit to the lover of your soul, it will become easier to obey His word and become an overcomer in this and every area of your life.

I am reminded of the Word of God. Some things take fasting and prayer to assist in prevailing over obstacles. Oh No, you say! More Denial! That's Discipleship! You don't fast to lose weight. You fast to improve your intimacy and relationship with God. Fasting will assist you, be beneficial, in the denial of carnal desires (Luke 21:34, Surfeiting: overindulgence in anything).

I can attest that fasting is a great tool. It has helped me. I suggest that you begin with the "Daniel fast". This fast consists of not eating meats, high carbohydrates, sweets, salty foods, sodas and such. Your body gets a vacation and is able to start the healing process. Not feeling bloated, sluggish, and weak should be a great incentive to changing your eating habits.

I found that after following the fast for a few weeks, a lot of food desires were diminished. I was a great coffee drinker; an all-day drinker: but now I find water is my thing. You will lose the desire for the health compromising foods and begin to yearn for the things that increase life and longevity.

You may decide that it's not that serious, your weight/health, but it certainly affects your life in areas seen and unseen. It will aid in your submission to God and enlighten you to knowing His purpose for you. He certainly desires for you to prosper and be in good Health, even as your soul prospers. Truly, if we want our "health to spring forth speedily (Isaiah 58:8), start with fasting a favorite drink or sweet dessert. Give up snacks. Even if you have to start slow, do something to jumpstart your body and prepare for transition.

Besides the health benefits of becoming healthier, wouldn't it be great not to buy anything with XL, W, Plus, or any of the Women's size adjectives? Being able to get closer to your husband would definitely get you points from him ladies, (comprende' vous?). You do understand, ladies?

Chapter Eight
Mind Over Matter

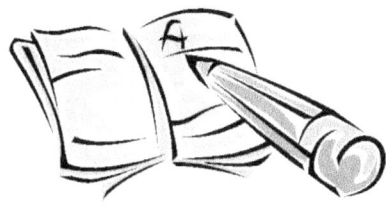 I would suggest that once you make up your mind, at least for 3 days, make a diary of how you eat. Record the when, why, time, and how you feel emotionally. This will give you a barometer to gauge real hunger or boredom or whatever it is that is causing you to overeat. Once you study your diary, you may find that it was not hunger, but other emotions that were ruling out of your soulish realm. Water satisfies thirst, not sodas. Sometimes we may feel we are hungry, but it may be thirst.

Drink some water! Water has such great properties. Light, refreshing, gets rid of toxins, aids digestion, and as a bonus, No calories. We should drink at least 8 glasses daily. Just drinking water can start the losing process. Put some lemon in your water, it helps intestinal cleansing and gives it some taste. I love diet Dr. Pepper, but sodas should be decreased or even eliminated during transition. Even though diet drinks have no calories, they do nothing for the body. I now drink a Dr. Pepper only once in a few weeks. Carbonation contributes to bloating and edema. They also contribute to the desire for sweets. Most sodas have high sugar and caloric count. Check out Coke, Sprite or Fanta. Some sodas have a high caffeine count which can affect medicinal effectiveness and may become addictive. Even diet sodas can keep the desire for sweets alive. Can you live without that double latte if it promotes new life?

The negative habits you developed will take about 30 days to break. By now, you are probably thinking," My coffee, my sodas, my whatever" (your overindulgence). Yes, you may go through withdrawal symptoms. I did! It didn't take very long, but I eventually no longer missed those things as much.

Yes, this may feel like you are nailing yourself to a cross and being crucified. You are! You are stopping the process of sickness and disease. The cycle is being broken. Even if you stop or somehow lose focus and motivation, jump right back on the road to Calvary's Hill. Loose your carnal man and begin to walk in your divinity. Walk into the new, better you!

Now for all you pretty young things! Perhaps, you can eat all you want now and suffer no unhealthy effects, but there is no age that cannot profit from a healthy lifestyle. Look at your gene pool! That's an indicator of what may become of you.

So, start now early in life and you will have lifelong benefits. If you are blessed with no health issues or weight problems and look Marvelous, be kind to your sisters and don't criticize. Bear them up! Your thing might not be food, but any and all desires work by the same self-spirit of lust. Enough said?

Chapter Nine

Made Up Mind

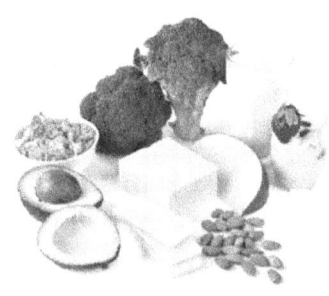 Next, let's look at color. Color! Yes! Eat nothing WHITE. I am not a dietician, but I have been a professional Eater! I knew what to eat and what food combination to produce the effect I needed at the time. Drug users, drinkers, smokers, and sexual permissive individuals do the same things to get "high". All is lust! It is the appetite (the spirit of the thing that is never satisfied).

No one wants to hurt or have pain or go through difficult circumstances. Eating it away only compounds the problem. It becomes a cycle filled with depression, despondency, and self-degradation. That's Not Healthy!

Even Jesus wanted his cup of suffering to go away. Propelled by purpose, He humbled himself and was obedient even to death. The only death here is to your carnal man and its works. Jesus gives the Spirit of Life and He gives you Joy!

White? The color white alerts me to kilocalories and things that convert to sugar. Bread, pasta, rice and certain comfort foods are such. Beware! Diabetics have to be very careful when consuming high carb (carbohydrates) foods.

Diabetics are auto-immune compromised. The body fights against itself. It does not recognize the insulin secreted by the pancreas or cannot utilize it correctly. This is Type II; Type I, your pancreas does not produce insulin at all. High carb foods convert to glucose.

What the body does not use stays in the bloodstream which produces havoc in every organ system in the body because the cardiovascular system supplies blood to every organ. Glucose filled blood is toxic and adverse to maintaining optimal and healthy vessels. High blood sugar contributes to stroke and heart disease. Decreased vision and neuropathy are also systematic of the disease.

Whole wheat toast rather than a biscuit is a great alternative for good low carbs and less calories over a biscuit with high carbs and high calories. Even if you have no health issue that warrants discipline, smart choices should be made and continued in every season of life.

There is such a great diversity of methods and choices that you can choose to assist in weight loss. Weight watchers has the highest success rate, but some praise Medifast, Sensa, and HCG hormone diets.

Perhaps, diet is a word that can be eliminated from your vocabulary. Let's say, that you are adopting a new healthy lifestyle. You can Google and be given a wealth of information and knowledge. I am sure you will find a system that will work for you. It must be a program that you can commit to.

Well, I've tried almost all of them. From the pills, the wraps, the fad diet, and the pay to lose pounds methods, that have worked temporarily. I didn't address the root cause. You cannot let things "eat"away at you. It is an everyday battle, even with my confession and success. By His stripes," I am Healed (Isa 55:3-5; I Peter 2:24)". Remember, the Lord is your Strength!

We are the Healed of the Lord and we do resist sickness and disease. Your affliction is the fruit of all your unresolved issues that have manifested in the extra weight. We conquer and prevail through His grace and mercy. He will deliver us out of our afflictions; give it to Him. His joy sustains.

48

Chapter Ten
A Green Mindset

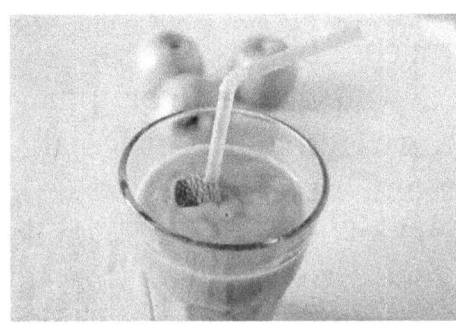 It has been said that we are what we eat. If you never eat your vegetables or salads and just indulge in fatty fried foods or high carb foods, you are heart attack bound. Green foods are healthy for you. Yes ladies, heart disease has become one of the top causes of death in women. Eat for strength and vigor.

Eat to live and not live to eat. You may not like veggies, but you can plan different ways to prepare them to make them tasty. Grilled veggies with a little olive oil and a sprinkling of sea salt, Yum! You can also do a power organic shake. Add spinach, kale, cucumber, coconut water, ginger, apple, carrots, flaxseed, cinnamon, and some mint and you have a good energy packed healthy drink to fuel you for your morning.

Here are a few suggestions that have been helpful to me:

- Start moving, walking gets the most benefits without impact; WALK IT OUT!
- Don't skip Breakfast (only if you are fasting), it's the most important meal. You will lessen spontaneous binges.
- Don't eat full, heavy meals after 6 or 7pm.
- Drink less coffee, try Herbal teas or Decaf.
- Instead of Ice Cream, eat Yogurt
- Try 2% milk, skim or even Soymilk, Almond milk is good also.
- Decrease sodas and carbonated drinks, color free sodas are more urinary tract friendly; it's the dyes.
- Take a multivitamin daily and/or supplements
- Use vinegar and lemon on salads rather than cream salad dressing, try Balsamic or Red wine vinegar.
- Use herbs and other seasonings and decrease salt. Salt promotes hunger and promotes edema, fluid retention.
- Have a veggie nite! Give your body a break from meats, especially red meat, eat red meat sparingly. It takes the body longer to digest. It just sits there.
- Bake, Broil, Grill, or Steam as an option from frying

- Avoid "white foods", go for the Green; veggies and fruits
- If a snack is needed, keep calorie count at 100 or below.
- Never shop if you are hungry. You will buy more junk food than good.
- Make your choices simple. If you like grilled chicken and salad every day, go for it. Go with what keeps you on track.
- Be consistent. Give your method a chance!
- After 2 weeks, if needed, give yourself a free day. Don't Binge, you will negate all the progress you have made.
- Boil Eggs;less calories. Try egg whites only
- Tuna, Salmon are low in calories and full of antioxidants.
- Have allowed snacks prepared and ready when hunger strikes
- No smoked meats! Try turkey and turkey bacon.
- Try whole wheat and whole grain rather than white bread or flour
- Try brown rice and wild rice instead of white rice
- Use wheat or veggie pasta
- Sweet potatoes rather than White potatoes, sparingly of course.
- Popcorn, Pork skins have no trans fat
- Yes, you could have had a V8, tomato juice is full of nutrients and low calorie

- The effects of exercise continue long after you stop. It keeps metabolizing
- Eat slower. It gives the brain time to tell your stomach it's full
- Use a smaller plate when fixing your food. This trains the eye to adopt smaller portions
- Do not eat less than 1000 calories daily. It has a negative impact on the body. Be wise! In fact, do not go below 1200 calories.
- It is better to eat 4 smaller low cal meals than go all day without eating and eat 2,000 calories at one sitting.
- Rest and sleep is important. This is the time the body uses to rejuvenate itself. If you never give it a break, it can not Heal itself.
- Stress is a fat producer. The stress hormone produces Cortisone (comes from Adrenal glands and inhibits metabolism). It manifests as extra fat and weight around the mid section. It loves your core, your center. It comes to steal your strength.
- Drink plenty of water, at least 8 glasses a day.
- Medium strawberries are about 6 calories per berry. The good thing is that you burn more calories to digest them.

- Try chicken, beef, or vegetable broth for an anytime light soup; add green onions and mushrooms. Yum!
- Read labels; you may be surprised at the sugar and salt content.
- Get enough rest; it is the body's time for rejuvenation.

Chapter Eleven
Masculine Mind

Men you are not excluded. Can I talk to you? You are our Kings and Priests. We love you and support you.

Although my target was to the women, I have found that the brothers who have read this book, have also benefitted. Kings, we want you to live forever. As head of our families, you lead and we follow. Our desire is that you be healthy and full of vim and vigor also.

Guys, how is your stamina? Where is your strength? You can tell the truth. Real men eat quiche, wear pink, cook dinner, have emotions, and sometimes even cry. Admit! That tire around your middle has no doubt compromised your prowess in significant areas of your life.

Your family may want to see you doing something other than clicking the remote. Can I tell you that heart disease is still the number one killer of men?   How is your blood pressure? How is your cholesterol?   Why am I messing with you Sons of Thunder?   I want you to live and have abundant life!

Psalms 91 let's us know that God is our Keeper; that He will deliver from the snare of the fowler (sickness, disease, heart problems, prostate, stoke, erectile dysfunction, dementia, and all afflictions).   None of these things will come nigh or near your dwelling place (your temple, His body) as a believer. He lives in you. You must take care of it!

I know it might be difficult to become vulnerable and admit to some things, but once you have addressed the issues of your heart, you can be healed and start to modify your eating habits.   You will begin to break the habitual overindulgence of health compromising foods.

I can see it now.   Its football season, actually any sport season, and you can be found in front of the TV with the remote in your hands, the chicken wings, the pizza, and the BBQ ribs are on the left. Your favorite drink is on the right, the recliner is at a 15 degree recline for optimal viewing, and you are ready for tip-off, kick-off, tee-off, face-off, batter-up, pole position or first serve. You are in your element! Am I right about it?

I must confess, that I am partial to sports too; especially tennis. What happens when one season is over; it overlaps to the next sport season. Therefore, non-movement, non-productivity and stagnancy is perpetuated. You get stuck! Get up from there! Move something other than hand to mouth. Change that cycle and circle.

Men, how can I tell that something is going on with you? It's not about watching sports. Enjoyment is not a bad thing. It's about the loss of motivation for the things of God and life that is manifesting in excess eating or drinking. Let's transfer your passion for sports into a passion for God and family. Rather, let God have the priority. Find His will and walk in it.

What is happening in your core? Your core is the excess baggage around your middle. The core is where your strength lives. Got muscles? Stress, anxiety, confusion, discouragement, and all emotional clutter abide in this area of the body. Cortisone is the stress hormone secreted by the adrenal glands; it combines with your poor eating habits and produces havoc in the digestive and endocrine systems.

Some of you may not be into sports, but the video games have a stronghold on you or you are a TV addict. Men love "Scandal" and "Soaps" too. It's ok! You are King!

I am sure that King David would not have been able to "have slain his thousands", if he was always eating at the priest's table. He had to stay fit and in shape. Saul's javelin would have killed him many of times, if he had not been swift of feet.

What javelin throws of the enemy are hitting its mark because you have no "quickening" to escape the tempter's fiery darts? We are behind you brothers, fathers, sons, husbands; we want you to be the best you can be and at your best. A healthy, tall or short, dark or light, handsome man with swagger! Yep! That's you!

Looking for a wife? A man that find a wife, find a good thing. Every thing that God made was good. Get rid of the tire, first. She may see it as a red flag and wonder about any unresolved issues. Got a wife? I am sure she would love getting closer to you at those special times. Get the lead out guys! Comprende'? You do understand? Right!

So, go back to the beginning and read the book. This time don't let your brain tell you it's a female thing. No, it's a healthy, live longer productive life thing. It begins with you changing your mindset.

Remember, God chose you to have dominion. What better way to demonstrate your kingship by having rule over your house; that is, your body. When you promote change, it will gravitate to the whole household. Kings, we want you to be strong and healthy. You are enabled to rule your kingdom. Are you ready to be transformed inside out? Ready, Set, Go; Read!

Men, did you know you have a slight advantage over women? Your metabolism works faster and burns more calories. You tend to lose weight at a faster pace. Men, you can cut out a few kilocalories and Boom, you are pounds thinner. Even if there are no physical demands on you (jobs, etc.), the benefits of a healthy, functioning mind and body is an added benefit of weight loss.

Sleep is sweet. Overeating can produce sleep, but no refreshing; just a bad, bloated feeling.

Instead of tossing and turning, you are able to sleep soundly and longer. You awaken refreshed and rejuvenated. Your body has had the chance to renew cells and produce energy. Congrats! You are becoming a new man. O King, Live forever!

Chapter Twelve

Be Aware, Be Mindful

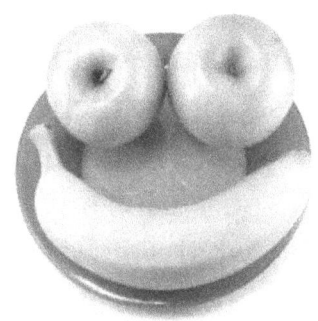 I have discussed many aspects of healthy living. It is important to be fully aware and informed concerning health care issues. Any addiction, whether food, prescription drugs, alcohol or smoking, all result in diminished health quality. You can reduce your risk by eliminating them from your lifestyle and adopting a different mindset.

2014 appeared to be a year wherein sickness and disease was rampant in our society. We are a people that are self-indulgent and physically weak. Over 50 million people will be diagnosed with Heart disease, Arthritis, Cancer, and Diabetes. We, as a people can change the statistics, one person at a time and one child at a time - beginning with you!

Let's look at these four major health concerns. God declares, *"He will heal our land"* II *Chronicles 7:14.* If we seek Him (inquire for help and strength) with our whole heart (turning away from unhealthy practices), he will hear and send healing (body, soul, and spirit). We do not have to settle or allow the enemy to steal our life. We are told in Psalms 91, that none of these things (sickness, disease, infirmities, or affliction) would come near our dwelling place. He is our assurance. So, if you are predisposed for any of these diseases, you can change what your gene pool has determined. You can be transformed in your inner man by changing what you put in your body.

Yes, it is challenging! You have to be consistent. I lost 60lbs by modifying my eating habits; and still became diabetic. My problem was that I did not get to the root of my over eating. I had done everything physically, but I did not allow the Word to plants new seeds of faith and perpetual healing in my inner man. The results were that I gravitated back to old mindsets. Now, I submit to the Word and allow it to perform surgery and removed all tentacles, links, and roots planted by the enemy. Hallelujah! Now, I agree with what the Word says and not what my emotions dictate. I gained 15lbs back while I was taking care of my elderly parents who were both extremely ill. No excuse. I took care of them and not myself. So, I had to get right back on track. I still have a long way to go, but I encouraged myself in the Lord. I lost those unwanted pounds and am working to continually be in alignment with the will of God; that is to be a Beautiful Blessed Woman.

Every age group, ethnicity, cultural, and socioeconomic people is under the attack. We must change the way we live and eat. Believers put on your armor. It is a daily battle. Persevere! We will continue to look at these killers of our society.

Heart disease or Cardiovascular disease, is the number one killer of men and women in America. Heart disease kills more women than breast cancer. This organ system controls the distribution of blood in the vessels of the body. It affects every other organ system. Even those that appear healthy may have cardiovascular problems. More common in males, but "A-fib" is one of the silent conditions that can cause stroke or heart attack anytime. A-fib for short is an electrical disruption in the pumping rhythm of the heart's upper chambers. Instead of a rhythmic collaboration with the lower ventricles, the Atria, flutters randomly at a high rate and blood flow weakens. Chronic A-fib weakens heart muscles. High blood pressure along with stress, alcohol, and a frantic lifestyle also contributes to this condition. Extreme exercise can cause a flutter and overwork the heart. Poor dental health and consistent jaw pain is also and indicator for cardiovascular problems.

Arthritis is a disease of the joints. Whether Rheumatoid or Osteoarthritis, it is very painful and can be debilitating. Osteoarthritis is caused by wear and tear on the joints. In advanced disease cases, the cartilage is completely gone and bone rubs against bone. 27 millions Americans are affected with this disease. There is no cure for Arthritis. The damage is great and the baby boomers are more affected than the previous generation. There are treatments that are diverse in their effectiveness. Also, there are treatments which are guided to reduce pain. It is primarily pain management rather than healing or cure that the doctors address.

They are:

1. Pills: pain pills increase the levels of serotonin and norepinephrine in the brain,

2. Injection medications are injected into the synovial fluid in joint spaces to relieve pain,

3. Distractions: this management involves placing a metal frame to distract the stress on a weakened joint, and

4.Cartilage replacement: involves getting cells from the cartilage and growing more cartilage to replace that which was lost. The doctors now try to reduce the more dramatic remedy of total joint replacement.

Cancer does not mean death. Again, millions of Americans have and will develop cancers. Whether breast, prostate, lung, colorectal, or blood cancers, you can work to reduce the percentage for you. You can eat to beat cancer. There are foods that reduce the risk of some cancers. Remember the "A Green Mindset" chapter? Look what a few foods can do!

1. **Apples**: Apples contain at least two kinds of cancer inhibiting compounds: flavonoids and phenolic acids.

2. **Nuts**: A serving of nuts, about a handful, wards off death from heart disease and cancer. Nuts also lower cholesterol levels.

3. **Beans and Lentils**: Loaded with fiber, beans and lentils contain antioxidants; phytochemicals and folate protect the colon. Soybeans may be helpful for treatment of prostate, lung, and colorectal cancers.

4. **Garlic and Onions**: these two pungent foods appear to stave off cancer by neutralizing carcinogenic (cancer making) substances and repairs damaged DNA.

5. **Milk**: the Calcium in diary products may neutralize potential carcinogens, particularly those found in processed meats. Milk drinkers are less likely to be obese also.

6. **Broccoli**: this green veggie is packed with sulforaphane; its cancer fighting substance is delivered to almost every tissue in the body.

7. **Tea and Coffee**: The antioxidants in coffee seem to be especially effective against endometrial cancer. Coffee lowers the risk of dementia by 65% if you drink 3-5 cups regularly; however, increased caffeine consumption is cautioned in those with cardiovascular

inclinations. Caffeine is addictive. Herbal organic teas are also good for you.

8. **Curry**: Curcumin, the main ingredient in the spice turmeric, fight against cancerous changes in healthy cells, also slows malignant cells.

9. **Tomatoes**: tomatoes are full of the antioxidant Lycopene. Tomatoes may block cancer by stopping the multiplication of malignant cells and cause them to destroy themselves.

10. **Dark Leafy Greens**: Arugula, Kale, Spinach, Romaine have abundant antioxidants called Carotenoids. They prohibit skin, lung, stomach, and some breast cancer cells.

11. **Red Grapes (Red wine):** grapes are loaded with Resveratrol which inhibits cancer-cell growth. It is also in peanuts, cranberries, and blueberries.

12. **Whole Grains**: 3-5 servings a day are linked to a lower risk of colorectal cancer. Whole grains protects against heart disease and Type II diabetes.

Diabetes has affected more than 25 million Americans. Losing weight, exercising daily and following a low fat diet, low carbs can reduce odds of getting the disease. If you are pre-disposed and have a family history of diabetes, it will be advantageous to adopt a healthier lifestyle. Here are some changes you might utilize to keep your blood sugar stable and prevent the onset of diabetes.

*Give up sodas: sugar sweetened soda increased risks of diabetes by 26%. The high fructose and caffeine can be addictive.

*Move after meals: take a 15-30 min stroll after you eat. This lowers post-meal blood sugar levels for at least 3 hours.

*Eat more good fat; adopting the Mediterranean lifestyle with the abundance of fish and olive oil, can lower risk of diabetes by 83%. Veggies, whole grains, and nuts lower blood sugar and cholesterol. Avocadoes are good fat.

*Get up already: sitting too long can be deadly. Extended sitting slows your body's ability to metabolize glucose.

* Bulk up: muscles are where you store most of your glucose (energy). Lifting weights can help release energy and strengthen muscles. Glucose

from food is released in blood and blood sugar rises if it is not utilized.

*Savor your food: Slow down and enjoy your food. Eating slowly increase satiety and prompts you to eat smaller portions.

Surround yourself with like minded people. The support will help you to stay on course. Knowing that these diseases are escalating should motivate you to adopt a healthier lifestyle. Prayer for temperance!

Conclusion

I pray that this book has encouraged you to continue pursing the abundant life that God has prepared for you. It is no secret that the thoughts that God has for you are good (Jer. 29:11). My prayer is that all the BBW will fulfill the potential and creative talents that are in them.

You are not alone and you can trust God. He is free and available! Allow yourself to be open again!

As mentioned before, when starting any weight loss journey, check with your doctor. There may be a medical condition that contributes to your weight loss challenges. Also, some medicines are compromised by different foods and/or juices. Once these issues are addressed and there is nothing to hinder you from becoming a healthier you, that is, only you: you can begin!

I hope you are motivated even as I am to becoming a stronger, energetic, and healthier woman. You can boldly proclaim, "He have delivered my soul in peace from the battle that was against me... (Psalms 55:18)". This goal lines up with God's purpose for every BBW (Blessed,

Beautiful, Woman). "Beloved, Above all things, I pray that you may prosper and be in Health even as thy soul prospers." I Celebrate you! Shalom!

KINGDOM KEYS TO MEDITATE UPON:

PSALMS 34:10, 42:11,103:5,145:18

_____
_____
_____
_____
_____

PROVERBS 10:11, 18:20, 23:1-3, 25:27-28,30:8

_____
_____
_____
_____
_____

ISAIAH 26:3.40:29

_____
_____
_____
_____
_____

PILLIPIANS 4:7

_____
_____
_____
_____
_____

HEBREWS 10:35

_____
_____
_____
_____
_____

Prayer

Father, in the name of Jesus, Thank you for revealing yourself to me. I am grateful for your faithfulness and your great mercy. Forgive me where I have missed you in this area of my life. Let me not be ruled by my carnal man with it lusts and desires.

Bind now the spirit of Lust, Over indulgence, Gluttony and Desire in me and Loose Temperance, Discipline, and Self-control in my life. Help me to mortify the deeds of my flesh and the lusts therein. My desire is for you and I submit myself to your plan and purpose. Give me strength to overcome and joy to sustain. Send the anointing power of the Holy Ghost to break every chain and fetter.

Let me walk in the spirit that I would not yield to the enemy and let my mouth be filled with your Word as my sword and defense. Let the cleansing power of the Blood purify and make me whole. Keep my heart and mind by your spirit and let nothing pollute the temple of God. Let my heart be filled with love by your spirit and keep me focus on you. Let me find rest in you as your kingdom is revealed in me. Father, I thank you and bless you. To you be glory and honor, dominion and power, forever, Amen.

_____

_____

_____

_____

_____

_____

_____

_____

_____

_____

_____

_____

_____

_____

_____

_____

_____

_____

_____

Inside Out

He's changing and transforming Me
Inside Out
I'm being made Free and full of victory
Inside Out
I'm finally becoming the real Me
Inside Out
I'm learning to let "it" all go
Inside out
Not afraid, I'm walking through the open door
Inside out
A new creation, gone is the negative of before
Inside Out
What's hidden can now be seen
Inside Out
Life is much fuller than I had ever dreamed
Inside Out
Now I can give glory and honor to the King
Inside Out
Without a doubt
Inside out
The battle was fought
Inside Out
I won the Peace that was Sought, Inside Out

Minister Deborah Ross

About the Author

Minister Deborah Ross is often called "Mom Ross". She is the mother and step-mother of ten children. Many children have come under her mentoring, nurturing, and care.

She is a native of Jacksonville, Florida where she resides. As a child, she was raised in eastern North Carolina and graduated from high school with honors.

Minister Ross is an anointed intercessor, exhorter, praise and worshipper, teacher, and scribe. She loves singing, dancing, cooking, writing, and most sports.

By profession, Deborah has worked over 25 yrs as a Radiologic Technologist, Phlebotomy technologist, and health care worker. She has won many awards and recognition in her field and has served on and held different state and local society offices.

She has an Associate's degree form Jacksonville theological Seminary for Christian Education as well as degrees in Health Care from Florida State College in Jacksonville, Florida.

Deborah is a award winner poet and has assisted other authors in their endeavors

Currently, she is connected to the capable leadership and dynamic ministry of Dr. Diane Clark, Kingdom Life Ministries, Itl., Jacksonville, FL 32218

Resources

Scripture Keys for Kingdom Living
Diabetic Management
Arthritis Today
Web MD.com
Vegetarian Cooking
Doctoroz.com/TV
AARP.com/magazine
Taber's Medical Cyclopedic Dictionary
Nelson's Reference Bible KJV/AMP